TRISHA LIZOTTE

Get Real

A Beginner's Guide to Choosing Real Food to Support Your Health

This book was professionally typeset on Reedsy.
Find out more at reedsy.com

"Let Food be Thy Medicine"

-HIPPOCRATES

Contents

1

Introduction

Welcome to Get Real, your introduction to real whole foods! In the busyness of life, it can be easy to overlook the importance of nourishing our bodies with wholesome, nutrient-dense foods. Oftentimes, we turn to processed, convenience foods that are high in sugar, salt, and unhealthy fats instead. While these foods may be convenient, they are making us obese and sick. It's time to change our mindset around what real food is and how it can help us live our best lives.

So what is "real" food? In this book, I will refer to real food, meaning whole food that is minimally processed and as close to its natural state as possible. They include fruits, vegetables, whole grains, lean proteins, and healthy fats. These foods are rich in essential vitamins, minerals, fiber, and antioxidants that our bodies need to function at their best. Food is meant to fuel your body and provide energy. In our world today, especially if you are reading this in America, we know that is not how we generally view or use food.

Incorporating these real foods into our diets has numerous health benefits. They can help us maintain a healthy weight, reduce our risk of chronic diseases such as heart disease and diabetes, improve our digestion, boost our energy levels, and even improve our mood, libido, and mental health. My goal in this book is to help you make conscious choices when it comes to what you put into your body and to show you how a few small changes can make you feel amazing. It's also important to recognize that we have so many alternatives available to us today to turn even our favorite comfort foods into healthier versions that support our goals.

In this book, you won't find an all-or-nothing approach when it comes to diet or nutrition. You also won't find me touting one fad diet or another or telling you to eliminate entire food groups. While I do believe it's better to avoid foods that make you feel bad, such as dairy if you are lactose intolerant, here we will explore the world of real whole foods in more detail to give a general understanding of why we need to add more real food to our diets. We will discuss the different types of whole foods, their nutritional benefits, and how to incorporate them into your diet in a practical and sustainable way. This book will provide you with the basic knowledge and tools you need to nourish your body with real, wholesome foods as you begin your wellness journey. So let's dive in and discover the amazing benefits of real whole foods!

2

Health Benefits of Real Whole Foods

Have you heard the term "garbage in, garbage out"? The food we eat is the fuel that powers our body. What we choose to eat has a significant impact on our overall health and well-being. Choosing nutrient-dense foods will provide the fuel needed to live an optimal life, lowering the risk of chronic diseases, improving digestion, helping with weight management, and increasing energy levels. When we choose foods that are highly processed, our bodies will not function at their best. That's when we start experiencing things like fatigue, moodiness, and unwanted gut issues.

Whole foods are packed with essential nutrients such as vitamins, minerals, fiber, and antioxidants that our body needs to function correctly and maintain optimal health. So, what are considered nutrient-dense foods? Foods in their most natural state such as fruits, vegetables, whole grains, and lean proteins provide a wide range of nutrients that can help prevent disease and improve overall health.

Diets rich in real whole foods have been shown to lower the risk of chronic diseases such as heart disease, diabetes, and some cancers.

These diseases are often referred to as lifestyle diseases because they are many times caused or contributed to by poor dietary habits, including consuming processed and refined foods that are high in sugar, unhealthy fats, and excessive sodium. Whole foods, on the other hand, are lower in calories and higher in nutrients, which can help prevent chronic diseases.

Whole Foods and Gut Health

Let's touch on a subject that has been making health headlines in recent years, gut health. If you struggle with a sluggish digestive system, IBS, leaky gut, or other uncomfortable digestive issues, adding whole foods to your diet is an important first step for improving digestion and overall gut health. These foods are high in fiber, which can help promote regular bowel movements and prevent constipation. Fiber also helps feed the good bacteria in our gut, which can improve gut health and boost the immune system. Increasing the amount of fruits, vegetables, whole grains, and legumes you consume can help significantly as these are excellent sources of fiber.

Keep in mind that when you begin adding these new foods to your diet, you may experience more intestinal discomfort at first. Your body needs time to adjust to this new way of eating. Don't get discouraged, it's very normal. There are products on the market designed to eliminate this issue that are readily available. I usually recommend products with the active ingredient simethicone.

Weight Management

Whole foods can also help with weight management. These foods are low in calories and high in nutrients, which can help us feel full and satisfied while consuming fewer calories. Whole foods are less processed and contain fewer unhealthy fats and sugars, which can contribute to weight gain. This is good news if you're like me and love to eat! In essence, you can eat more, stay fuller longer, and be healthier.

Fatigue

Do you struggle with fatigue? Whole foods can help increase energy levels. These foods are high in nutrients that our body needs to produce energy, such as complex carbohydrates, protein, and healthy fats. Whole foods are less processed and contain fewer unhealthy additives that can contribute to fatigue. Instead of grabbing that extra cup of coffee or sugary snack, try eating an apple with nut butter when you feel an energy slump.

Libido

Eating a healthy diet can also have a positive impact on libido. Whole foods are rich in nutrients that can help improve blood flow, reduce inflammation, and support hormone production, all of which can contribute to a healthier sex drive. For example, foods high in antioxidants, such as berries and dark chocolate, can help improve blood flow and reduce inflammation in the body, which can improve sexual function. Additionally, foods high in zinc, such as oysters and pumpkin seeds, can help support healthy testosterone levels, which can also contribute to a healthy libido. By incorporating these foods into your diet, you may notice an improvement in your overall sexual health and well-being. You're welcome!

Sleep

Eating a healthy diet filled with whole foods can also have a significant impact on sleep quality. Whole foods are naturally rich in nutrients that can help regulate our sleep-wake cycle and promote better sleep. Foods high in magnesium, such as dark leafy greens and nuts, can help relax the muscles and promote sleep. Additionally, foods high in tryptophan, such as turkey and bananas, can help increase the production of serotonin, a neurotransmitter that regulates sleep. On the other hand, consuming processed and high-sugar foods can disrupt our sleep by causing blood sugar spikes and crashes.

Hormones

While this is not a book on hormone health and I am not a hormone expert, it is proven that hormones are greatly affected by what we eat. Whole foods can have a significant positive impact on our hormones. Eating a diet rich in whole foods such as the ones mentioned in this book can help regulate hormones such as insulin, cortisol, and estrogen. These foods contain essential vitamins, minerals, and fiber that support healthy hormone function. On the other hand, processed and refined foods, high in sugar and unhealthy fats, and even diet soda can wreak havoc on hormone balance and lead to inflammation in the body. Incorporating whole foods into your diet can not only improve your overall health, but also positively impact your hormonal health. As we age, especially women who are in perimenopause or menopause, it is even more crucial to understand how what we eat affects our hormones. There are many good resources available that go deeper into that subject, however, always consult with your doctor if you have concerns.

3

Whole Food - Keeping it Simple

As mentioned, eating real whole foods is one of the best ways to maintain a healthy lifestyle. Whole foods are nutrient-dense and provide the body with essential vitamins, minerals, and fiber. This chapter will discuss some of the most common examples of real whole foods and their correlating health benefits.

Fruits and vegetables are some of the most important whole foods. They are packed with nutrients, fiber, and antioxidants that help protect the body against disease. Some examples of low-sugar fruits and vegetables include:

- Apples
- Berries
- Citrus fruits
- Leafy greens
- Cruciferous vegetables (broccoli, cauliflower, kale)
- Tomatoes

Whole grains are an excellent source of fiber, protein, and complex carbohydrates. Let's dispel the myth that all carbs are bad. Carbs are not the enemy. They are an essential source of energy for the body. They are also rich in vitamins and minerals. Reducing or eliminating simple carbs that turn to sugar, such as white bread, white rice, and white pasta, can positively impact our health. While incorporating some of these healthier complex carbohydrates below will help your body be more efficient in using those calories as energy.

- Brown rice
- Quinoa*
- Oats
- Barley
- Whole wheat bread
- Whole grain pasta

*Quinoa is a grain that is also a complete protein. In other words, it has all the amino acids that would be contained in animal proteins but is plant-based. Quinoa is a great source of protein if you are trying to eliminate or reduce your intake of animal protein.

Nuts and seeds are an excellent source of healthy fats, protein, and fiber. They are also rich in vitamins and minerals. Nuts and seeds make a great snack or salad topping. Try adding some of the following to your diet regularly:

- Almonds
- Walnuts
- Cashews
- Chia seeds
- Flaxseeds
- Pumpkin seeds

Legumes are a good source of protein, fiber, and complex carbohydrates. They are also rich in vitamins and minerals. Legumes include:

- Lentils
- Chickpeas
- Black beans
- Kidney beans
- Peas
- Soybeans

Plant-based proteins are an excellent alternative to animal proteins. They are low in saturated fat and high in fiber. Some examples of plant-based proteins include:

- Tofu
- Tempeh
- Seitan (made from gluten, so avoid if you are gluten intolerant)
- Lentils
- Chickpeas
- Black beans
- Quinoa

Lean proteins are an essential part of a healthy diet. They are low in saturated fat and provide the body with essential nutrients. Some examples of lean proteins include:

- Chicken breast
- Turkey breast
- Fish (salmon, tuna, cod)
- Lean beef (filet mignon, sirloin)
- Eggs

Healthy fats are an essential part of a healthy diet. They help maintain healthy skin, hair, and nails. Some examples of healthy fats include:

- Avocado
- Olive oil
- Coconut oil
- Nuts and seeds
- Fatty fish (salmon, tuna, mackerel)

Eating whole foods is one of the best ways to maintain a healthy lifestyle. Incorporating a variety of fruits and vegetables, whole grains, nuts and seeds, legumes, plant-based proteins, lean proteins, and healthy fats into your diet can provide the body with essential nutrients and help protect against disease. By making some of these small suggested changes to your diet, you can significantly improve your overall health.

4

Tips for Incorporating Whole Foods into Your Diet

Incorporating whole foods into your diet can seem like a daunting task, especially if you are used to eating processed and packaged foods. However, it is important to make this change for the sake of your health. Whole foods are those that are minimally processed and do not contain added sugars, preservatives, or artificial ingredients. Recall these are nutrient-dense foods and provide the body with the necessary vitamins, minerals, and fiber it needs to function properly. In this chapter, we will discuss five tips for incorporating more whole foods into your diet.

Start small and gradually increase intake:
One of the biggest mistakes people make when trying to switch to a whole foods diet is trying to do it all at once. This can be overwhelming and unsustainable. Instead, start small by incorporating one or two whole foods into your diet each week. For example, you could start by adding a serving of fresh fruit to your breakfast or swapping out your afternoon salty snack for a handful of nuts. As you become more comfortable with these changes, gradually increase your intake of whole

foods until they make up the majority of your diet.

Experiment with new recipes and flavors:
Eating whole foods does not have to be boring or tasteless. There are countless recipes and flavor combinations to explore. Try experimenting with new recipes and ingredients to keep your meals interesting and flavorful. You could try making a vegetable stir-fry with a variety of colorful veggies, or a hearty salad with mixed greens, roasted vegetables, and a homemade vinaigrette.

Plan meals and snacks to avoid common pitfalls:
One of the biggest challenges of eating a whole foods diet is avoiding common pitfalls like fast food and processed snacks. To avoid these temptations, it is important to plan your meals and snacks. This could involve meal prepping for the week ahead or packing healthy snacks to take with you on the go. By having healthy options readily available, you are less likely to reach for unhealthy alternatives.

Shop the perimeter of the grocery store:
When shopping for whole foods, it is important to focus on the perimeter of the grocery store. This is where you will find fresh produce, meats, and dairy products. The center aisles are typically filled with processed and packaged foods that should be mostly avoided. You will, however, find your beans, whole grain rice, pasta, quinoa, dried herbs and spices in these aisles. But you get the point. By shopping the perimeter, you can ensure that you are filling your cart with whole, nutrient-dense foods that will support your goals.

Choose minimally processed options:
When selecting whole foods, it is important to choose minimally processed options. This means opting for fresh fruits and vegetables

(frozen is fine too), whole grains, and lean proteins. Opt for more plant-based proteins over animal proteins which are harder to digest. Avoid foods that are heavily processed or contain added sugars, preservatives, or artificial ingredients. By choosing minimally processed options, you can ensure that you are getting the most nutrients and health benefits from your food.

Incorporating whole foods into your diet can be a challenging but rewarding process. By starting small, experimenting with new recipes, planning meals and snacks, shopping the perimeter of the grocery store, and choosing minimally processed options, you can make the transition to a whole foods diet more manageable. Remember to be patient with yourself and celebrate small wins along the way. With time and dedication, you can achieve your health and wellness goals.

5

Cooking Methods

Healthy cooking methods are an essential part of this journey to maintaining a nutritious diet and reducing the risk of chronic diseases. Some of the best cooking methods for healthy eating include steaming, grilling, and baking. Additionally, using non-stick cookware and avoiding deep-frying can also help to reduce the amount of added fats and oils used in your meals.

Grilling is a healthy way to cook lean meats and fish, as it allows excess fat to drip away. I also love to put all my spring/summer veggies on the grill.

Baking/roasting is another great option for cooking meats and vegetables, as it requires little to no added fat.

Steaming can be a good option for cooking vegetables, as it preserves their natural flavors and nutrients as long as you only cook them al dente.

Do you love fried food? Ahhh, me too! But, I don't love all the unhealthy fats and oils that go along with it. I found a solution to that! I use my air fryer almost every day. I air fry potatoes, veggies, fish, chicken, you name it! If you don't have an air fryer, I highly recommend you get one. It will help you immensely in your journey. Seriously, it's so good with none of the oil! Best of all, it's so easy to use even if you can't cook or don't like to cook!

By incorporating these healthy cooking methods into your daily routine, you can enjoy delicious and nutritious meals that are good for your body and mind.

6

Alcohol

Let's talk about alcohol briefly. Personally, I am not much of a drinker, but I also do not demonize alcohol. Alcohol has both pros and cons when it comes to health. On the positive side, moderate alcohol consumption, mainly red wine, has been linked to a reduced risk of cardiovascular disease, as it can increase levels of HDL (good) cholesterol and decrease the risk of blood clot formation. Additionally, some studies have found that moderate alcohol consumption may have a protective effect against certain cancers, such as colon and breast cancer. However, excessive alcohol consumption can have serious negative effects on health, including liver damage, high blood pressure, and an increased risk of certain cancers. It can also lead to addiction and mental health issues such as depression and anxiety. Overall, it is important to consume alcohol in moderation and be aware of the potential risks to our health. If weight loss is your goal, you will want to reduce your alcohol intake to no more than 3-4 ounces and one to two times per week or eliminate it completely.

If you are trying to eliminate or cut back on your alcohol consumption, but find yourself in social situations where you would normally have a cocktail, try one of these delicious mocktails from Oprah Daily instead. You won't even miss the alcohol...or the hangover!

Baby Bellini
Enjoy this chic and delicate mocktail over brunch
Ingredients:

- 2 ounces peach nectar
- 4 to 5 ounce sparkling cider
- Peach slice

Instructions:
Pour peach nectar into a champagne glass, then add the sparkling cider. Garnish with the peach slice.

Cos-Mock

Love a good cosmo? This mocktail will not only taste like the original, it will provide a dose of vitamin C
Ingredients (2 servings):

- ¼ cup Seville orange marmalade
- Juice of 1 lime
- ½ cup cranberry juice
- Lemon twists

Instructions:
Place marmalade in a strainer over a small bowl. Add 2 Tbsp. boiling water while forcing the jelly, not peels, through the strainer. Stir it in the bowl. Place this marmalade syrup in a mixing glass. Add the lime juice, cranberry juice, ice, then stir. Serve in two cocktail glasses with

the lemon twists to finish it off.

7

Water

You didn't think I would write a nutrition guide and not include a chapter on water, did you? While not technically food, water plays a vital role in maintaining overall health and wellness. I know you probably hear it all the time, but the truth is water is often overlooked as a crucial component of a healthy diet. Our bodies are made up of approximately 60% water, and it is essential for many of our bodily functions.

One of the most important roles of water is to help regulate body temperature. Without enough water, our bodies cannot effectively regulate our temperature, which can lead to overheating and dehydration.

Water is also important for digestion and nutrient absorption. It helps to break down food and transport nutrients throughout the body. Without enough water, our digestive system can become sluggish, leading to constipation and other uncomfortable digestive issues. Start your day with an 8-ounce glass of room-temperature lemon water before grabbing that first cup of coffee. This will wake your digestive system and rehydrate you after a night of sleep.

And bonus…drinking enough water can also help to improve skin health. When our bodies are dehydrated, our skin can become dry and dull. Drinking plenty of water helps to keep our skin hydrated and can even help to reduce the appearance of wrinkles. If that's not motivation enough, in addition to these benefits, drinking enough water can also help to boost energy levels, improve cognitive function, and support kidney function. Whenever I sense the onset of a headache or fatigue early in the day, I make it a point to assess my water intake, which often turns out to be much less than I assumed. Boosting my intake of water almost always eases my symptoms and revitalizes me.

So how much water should you be drinking? The general recommendation is to drink at least 8 eight ounces glasses of water per day, but this varies depending on age, weight, and activity level. I encourage my clients to drink at least half their body weight in ounces of water each day. It's important to listen to your body and drink water whenever you feel thirsty. Here's an interesting fact - sometimes we mistake thirst for hunger. The next time you feel hungry for a snack, try drinking eight ounces of water first and see if the urge goes away.

If you have trouble drinking enough water throughout the day, try adding some fresh fruit (lemons or berries) or cucumbers to add flavor. You can also fill the number of water bottles needed to reach your goal and keep them in the refrigerator so that you know when you have finished drinking the last bottle, you have met your daily intake goal.

8

Supplements

I receive many, many requests for recommendations on supplements. There is not a one size fits all answer. No two people are exactly alike and our needs are different. The simple answer is most everyone can benefit from a multivitamin. Even the healthiest eaters among us likely do not get all the vitamins and minerals we need through our food, mostly due to how our food is grown in soil that has been degraded. Consider it like a little insurance that you are ensuring you are reaching your minimal daily values. The best way to know what you need is to have your doctor or functional nutritionist run your labs. They can then help you ensure you are only taking what you need for your unique situation.

One recommendation I will make confidently is digestive enzymes. If you are introducing vegetables to your diet for the first time or increasing the number of fruits and vegetables you are eating, you very likely could experience some issues in the beginning. Increased gas and bloating are very common until your body adjusts to this new way of eating. Digestive enzymes can help your body process these foods more easily and make you more comfortable. I always keep them on hand. Cooking your vegetables instead of eating them raw can also help with digestion.

9

Let's Get Real

I know change is hard! But...if you didn't want to change, you wouldn't be reading this book. So here we are. The title of this book is Get Real. While the title is referring primarily to food, I would be doing you a disservice if I didn't provide just a bit of tough love and encouragement to get real with yourself.

Why do you want to make this change? Is it to prevent or reverse disease? Lose weight? Improve overall health? Be an example for your kids? Without answering this question, it will be unlikely to create sustainable change, no matter how many books you read on nutrition.

After studying nutrition for almost two decades, I have coached hundreds of people on mindset and lifestyle changes. I understand firsthand how difficult it can be to change habits so deeply ingrained in us that they have become part of our identity. What is that internal dialogue you are having right now? I urge you to be so sick and tired of feeling sick and tired that you tell yourself failure is not an option this time. When you fall, you get back up. Stop making excuses and convincing yourself that it's too hard to change. Change is tough, but so are you.

This is not about a diet! Please remove that word from your vocabulary. It's a toxic word that has too many negative connotations to use in your health journey. I am teaching you how to slowly improve your health by creating a sustainable lifestyle that will dramatically improve every aspect of your life. You see, this body that you are in today is the only body you get. When your health is failing, your quality of life is directly impacted. When you have your health, everything else falls into place. Being a healthier person in mind, spirit and body will make you a better partner, parent, employee, and friend and you have more to give to this world. You are free to be the best version of YOU!

10

Bonus Material

Recipe Ideas and Easy Swaps
Try these simple whole-food recipes that are both nutritious and delicious:

Avocado Toast with Poached Egg
Ingredients:

- 1 slice of whole grain bread
- 1/2 ripe avocado
- 1 egg
- 1 tsp white vinegar
- Salt and pepper to taste

Instructions:

1. Toast the bread until it is crispy.
2. While the bread is toasting, cut the avocado in half and remove the pit. Scoop out the flesh and mash it with a fork in a small bowl.
3. Bring a pot of water to a boil and add the white vinegar.

4. Crack the egg into a small bowl or ramekin.

5. Reduce the heat of the pot to a simmer and gently pour the egg into the water. Use a spoon to shape the egg whites around the yolk.

6. Cook the egg for about 3 minutes, or until the whites are set and the yolk is still runny.

7. Remove the egg from the water with a slotted spoon and place it on a paper towel to drain.

8. Spread the mashed avocado on the toast and sprinkle with salt and pepper.

9. Top the avocado with the poached egg and sprinkle with additional salt and pepper if desired.

Quinoa Salad with Roasted Vegetables

Ingredients:

- 1 cup of cooked quinoa*
- 1 red bell pepper, sliced
- 1 zucchini, sliced
- 1/2 red onion, sliced
- 2 tbsp olive oil
- 1 garlic clove, minced
- Salt and pepper to taste
- Handful of fresh spinach leaves
- 1/4 cup of crumbled feta cheese (optional but delicious!)

Instructions:

- Preheat the oven to 400°F (200°C).
- In a large bowl, toss the sliced bell pepper, zucchini, and red onion with olive oil, minced garlic, salt, and pepper.

- Spread the vegetables out on a baking sheet and roast in the oven for 20-25 minutes, or until they are tender and slightly browned.
- In a separate bowl, combine the cooked quinoa with the roasted vegetables.
- Add a handful of fresh spinach leaves and crumbled feta cheese to the quinoa and vegetables.
- Toss everything together until well combined.
- Serve the quinoa salad warm or chilled.

Grilled Salmon with Roasted Vegetables

Ingredients:

- 4 salmon filets
- 1 lemon, sliced
- 1 tbsp olive oil
- Salt and pepper to taste
- 2 cups of mixed vegetables (such as broccoli, carrots, and sweet potatoes)
- 2 tbsp balsamic vinegar
- 1 tbsp honey
- 1 garlic clove, minced
- Salt and pepper to taste

Instructions:

- Preheat the grill to medium-high heat.
- Brush the salmon filets with olive oil and season with salt and pepper.
- Place the salmon filets on the grill and top each filet with a slice of lemon.
- Grill the salmon for 5-7 minutes on each side, or until it is cooked

through.

- While the salmon is grilling, preheat the oven to 400°F (200°C).
- Toss the mixed vegetables with balsamic vinegar, honey, minced garlic, salt, and pepper.
- Spread the vegetables out on a baking sheet and roast in the oven for 20-25 minutes, or until they are tender and slightly browned.
- Serve the grilled salmon with the roasted vegetables.

You don't have to skip dessert. Remember, in this book, we are not talking about deprivation or even weight loss. The goal of this book is to incorporate more real whole foods into your diet consistently.

Healthier version of your favorite desserts

For the Love of Chocolate Brownies
Ingredients:

- 1 cup almond flour (coconut flour can be substituted)
- 1/2 cup cocoa powder
- 1/2 cup honey
- 1/2 cup unsweetened applesauce
- 2 eggs (or equivalent egg replacement)
- 1 tsp vanilla extract
- 1/2 tsp baking soda
- 1/2 cup dark chocolate chips

Instructions:

1. Preheat your oven to 350°F (175°C) and grease an 8x8 inch baking dish with cooking spray.

2. In a large mixing bowl, whisk together the almond flour, cocoa powder, and baking soda.
3. In a separate bowl, whisk together the honey, applesauce, eggs, and vanilla extract.
4. Add the wet ingredients to the dry ingredients and stir until well combined.
5. Fold in the dark chocolate chips.
6. Pour the batter into the prepared baking dish and smooth out the top with a spatula.
7. Bake for 20-25 minutes or until a toothpick inserted into the center comes out clean.
8. Let the brownies cool for at least 10 minutes before slicing and serving.

Enjoy your delicious and healthy chocolate brownies!

We love this **no-bake chocolate pudding** recipe:
Ingredients:

- 1 ripe avocado
- 1/4 cup unsweetened cocoa powder
- 1/4 cup honey or maple syrup
- 1/4 cup almond milk
- 1 tsp vanilla extract
- Pinch of salt

Instructions:

1. Cut the avocado in half and remove the pit. Scoop the flesh into a blender or food processor.
2. Add the cocoa powder, honey or maple syrup, almond milk, vanilla

extract, and salt to the blender or food processor.

3. Blend all the ingredients until smooth and creamy.
4. Pour the mixture into small serving bowls or glasses.
5. Chill in the refrigerator for at least 30 minutes before serving.
6. Enjoy your guilt-free, healthy chocolate dessert!

I scream, you scream, we all scream for NICE cream

Check out our favorite super simple dairy-free version of Chunky Monkey ice cream recipe:

Ingredients:

- 1 tbsp of plant milk (add more as needed)
- ½ frozen banana
- 1 tsp peanut or other nut butter
- Vegan chocolate chips

Instructions:

1. Small handful of ice into food processor high speed blender
2. Add plant milk, banana and nut butter to blender
3. Blend until smooth
4. Top with vegan chocolate chips and enjoy!

Easy Swaps to Stay on Track

It's not easy giving up some of our favorite foods, but when we can find healthier options to replace them, we aren't giving them up at all! I don't believe in deprivation and I am a self-declared french fry addict. I am always on the hunt for a more natural alternative to my favs.

Here is a list of some healthy food swaps for unhealthy foods for quick reference:

Unhealthy Food ➡ Healthy Swap

Potato chips ➡ Baked or airfried kale chips, homemade baked or airfried corn tortilla chips

White bread ➡Whole grain bread

Soda (including diet soda) ➡Flavored natural sparkling water

Ice cream ➡Frozen yogurt, fruit sorbet or our nice cream recipe listed above

French fries ➡ Baked or airfried sweet potato fries, homemade baked or airfried fries

Candy ➡ Fresh fruit or dried fruit

Fried chicken ➡ Grilled, baked or airfried chicken

Pizza ➡Homemade pizza with whole wheat crust and veggies

Processed snacks ➡ Nuts or seeds

Sugary cereal ➡ Oatmeal with fresh berries or nuts

Remember, making small changes to your diet can have a big impact on your overall health and well-being. If you need more help with swaps, follow me on Insta and check out my bio for free resources.

11

Conclusion

We have explored the many benefits of eating real whole foods and the positive impact on our health and well-being. By choosing to incorporate more whole foods into our diet, we can improve our digestion, boost our immune system, balance our hormones, and reduce our risk of chronic diseases.

While it may seem daunting to completely overhaul our eating habits, it's important to remember that small changes can make a big difference. Start by incorporating one or two whole foods into your meals each day, such as swapping out processed snacks for fresh fruit or adding more vegetables to your plate.

As a health coach, I want to encourage you to set achievable goals for yourself and celebrate your progress along the way. Remember that a healthy diet is not about perfection, but about making progress towards a more balanced and nourishing lifestyle. With commitment and consistency, you can achieve your wellness goals and live your best life.

So let's commit to prioritizing our health and well-being by choosing real whole foods and making small changes towards a healthier diet. Your body will thank you for it.

If you found this book helpful, I would be very appreciative if you would leave the book a favorable review on Amazon.

12

Resources

Dreher M, Davenport AJ. (2013). Avocado consumption is associated with better diet quality and nutrient intake, and lower metabolic syndrome risk in US adults. *National Health and Nutrition Examination Survey.* https://doi.org/10.1186/1475-2891-12-1

Wang, X., Ouyang, Y., Liu, J., Zhu, M., Zhao, G., Bao, W., & Hu, F. B. (2014). Fruit and vegetable consumption and mortality from all causes, cardiovascular disease, and cancer: systematic review and dose-response meta-analysis of prospective cohort studies. *BMJ, 349*(jul29 3), g4490. https://doi.org/10.1136/bmj.g4490

Position of the American Dietetic Association: Health Implications of Dietary Fiber. (2008). *Journal of the American Dietetic Association, 108*(10), 1716–1731. https://doi.org/10.1016/j.jada.2008.08.007

Mozaffarian, D., Hao, T., Rimm, E. B., Willett, W. C., & Hu, F. B. (2011). Changes in Diet and Lifestyle and Long-Term Weight Gain in Women and Men. *The New England Journal of Medicine, 364*(25), 2392–2404.

RESOURCES

https://doi.org/10.1056/nejmoa1014296

Harvard T.H. Chan School of Public Health. (2017). Healthy Eating Plate. Retrieved from https://www.hsph.harvard.edu/nutritionsour ce/healthy-eating-plate/. *harvard.edu.* Retrieved June 8, 2023, from https://www.hsph.harvard.edu/nutritionsource/healthy-eating-plate /

mayo clinic. (2021). *Whole grains: Hearty options for a healthy diet. Retrieved from https://www.mayoclinic.org/healthy-lifestyle/nutrition-an d-healthy-eating/in-depth/whole-grains/art-20047826.* Retrieved June 8, 2023, from https://www.mayoclinic.org/healthy-lifestyle/nutrition-a nd-healthy-eating/in-depth/whole-grains/art-20047826

Protein foods. (2021). *Retrieved From https://www.niddk.nih.gov/he alth-information/weight-management/tips-getting-active/protein-foods.* https://www.niddk.nih.gov/health-information/weight-managemen t/tips-getting-active/protein-foods

Vinuales, L. (2023, January 3). 27 Best Mocktail Recipes for When You Want a Break from Alcohol. *Oprah Daily.* https://www.oprahdaily.com /life/g38744562/best-mocktail-recipes/